The Ketogenic Diet

Boost Your Metabolism, Burn the Fat and
Lose Weight Fast Living the Ketogenic Lifetyle

Sara Elliott Price

Published in The USA by:

Success Life Publishing

125 Thomas Burke Dr.

Hillsborough, NC 27278

Copyright © 2015 by Sara Elliott Price

ISBN-10: 151187242X

Disclaimer

Every effort has been made to accurately represent this book and its potential. Results vary with every individual, and your results may or may not be different from those depicted. No promises, guarantees or warranties, whether stated or implied, have been made that you will produce any specific result from this book. Your efforts are individual and unique, and may vary from those shown. Your success depends on your efforts, background and motivation.

The material in this publication is provided for educational and informational purposes only and is not intended as medical advice. The information contained in this book should not be used to diagnose or treat any illness, metabolic disorder, disease or health problem. Always consult your physician or health care provider before beginning any nutrition or exercise program. Use of the programs, advice, and information contained in this book is at the sole choice and risk of the reader.

Table of Contents

Introduction

The Ketogenic diet has been in existence officially in western medicine since the 1920's, but knowledge of the science behind it dates back to ancient Greece. Limit the consumption of sugars, trigger the creation of ketones cause the body and brain to use fats instead of sugars. That's the process in a nutshell.

Following the diet means eating a lot of natural fats, eating a little protein, and holding the carbs. Strictly sticking with it causes healthy weight loss, stopping seizures in epileptic seizure sufferers, some studies even show a possible slowing of cancer growth, and a myriad of other health benefits.

It's important to consult a doctor before starting this diet, as the processes it sets forth in the body are powerful and sufferers of certain conditions might find this inappropriate, or even harmful. Monitoring the presence of ketonic bodies is an essential part of the experience, so make sure you contact your doctor.

Use this book as a guide, inspiration and road map, but your doctor is the authority. Make sure you respect that before setting out and trying the diet.

That said, it's really a simple lifestyle change that can turn your health around for the better. Some willpower and motivation are what you need to make it happen.

Chapter 1:
Stepping Into the Ketogenic Diet

The Ketogenic diet is a great way to improve health and reduce pain. It is also a fabulous way to lose weight, to look and feel great. An overall feeling of well-being is prevalent, the pounds fall off and your dream weight is achieved. Finally: a diet that really works.

The Ketogenic diet was originally designed to stop epileptic seizures. It is so effective that when followed strictly, it eliminates the need for anti-seizure drugs and other invasive procedures.

The diet is not just one of many low-carb diets. It is a heavy-duty fat burning tool. The amazing part? You get to eat lots of (natural source) fat. The proportions of 75% fat, 20% protein and 5% carbohydrate is essential. The reason lies in the processes that this combination and balance causes the body to undertake.

Sugars, carbohydrates and starches are broken down as glucose in the bloodstream. Normally, the body uses this glucose for fuel. But glucose is also often poison to the body, as diabetics often experience. Glucose not only fuels normal bodily processes, it feeds cancer. Cancer cells get their energy via fermentation, and glucose is needed for fermentation to take place. Studies have shown that if you starve the cancer cells of glucose, the cancer can be treated more effectively.

Because fat is a more efficient source of energy than sugar in the body, athletes looking to perform better and achieve more lean bodies often turn to this diet. With resources such as this very book now in abundance, it is easy to put the diet into practice.

People who have tried the diet and adhered to the standards have reported not feeling hungry (like they often do with other, less effective diets) and have found it easy to follow the guidelines and recipes. If you've ever tried the Atkins diet, or the Paleo diet, then a lot of the concepts, recipes and ideas will be familiar to you.

Let's look at a brief history of the Ketogenic diet. Back in the 1920's, it was found that limiting carbohydrates stops seizures in sufferers of epileptic seizures. This was the prescribed method of treatment, and it was extremely successful. However, later, as anti-seizure drugs arose, the diet was forgotten.

Then Hollywood director Jim Abrahams re-discovered the diet when desperately searching for a way to help his epileptic son Charlie, who was 2 years old at the time. After failed attempts with medication and invasive surgery, Abrahams was ready to try anything. The family was astounded and delighted when after a month, Charlie's seizures totally stopped. He remained on the diet for years, and his condition healed completely. Abrahams even made a film called First Do No Harm (starring Meryl Streep) based on his family's experience, and to help others in a similar position find out that there are options out there. As the public became aware of this story, others reached for the diet for better health and increased weight loss.

This book is a practical guide to getting on the diet and staying on it. It gets into various reasons for going on the diet, and which health conditions can be improved with it. We will discuss some of the science behind why this works, and what happens when your body is in a ketonic state. We'll see which foods we can eat, in what amounts and with which other foods they can be eaten with. Finally, there will be some handy and delicious recipes for you to try, followed by some tips for motivation and inspiration.

Above all, you must have the will to improve your health, look and feel great and live up to your potential. Here's an opportunity to make a big change for the better in your life. You will alter the way you eat, and also the way you think about food. Your awareness about food and other aspects of your life will come into focus. Many people who failed in every other diet they had ever tried have lost significant amounts of weight, without EVER feeling hungry. (Because you get to eat lots of fat, you will be satiated. Your body will in turn use this fat, and your body will look lean, and you will feel great). You can do this too.

Chapter 2:
What are Ketones and How Do They Aid Weight Loss?

Ketones are the metabolic product of fat burning, which arise in the body when carbohydrate intake is strictly limited. The body can run on glucose or on ketones. When there isn't any sugar to process, the body produces ketones in response to a low insulin environment. The lowered insulin allows the body to access fat deposits as fatty acids flow into the liver. Fat is then burned, and extra fat deposits are used up. (In a typical high carb diet, the glucose is used first, whereas whatever fat that is consumed gets stored on the body).

To put it simply, ketones are the alternative fuel source your body uses if there isn't any glucose there for it to run on. A common misconception out there is that the body NEEDS glucose. Not so. This is perhaps justification for the way most people eat, which is very heavy on breads, noodles, pastries, candies, soda and the like. It's not healthy, nor is it efficient. It also causes the body to send hunger signals when it doesn't need to feed more. (What we all need more of is nutrition, and we can get more of this by eating healthy fats like coconut oil and eating leafy greens in the context of the ketogenic diet).

So, the presence of ketones means there is a lack of glucose and insulin. (This is because the body doesn't need the insulin to transport the glucose to use as fuel). This is good for normal cells, as their optimal energy source can now be used. It is bad for cancer cells, since they need glucose for fermentation, which is the only way they can get energy. This is an excellent way to possibly slow the growth of cancer, or to prevent it in the first place!

To get the body to this optimal fat-burning state, we need to reduce carbs to a very small amount. This means cutting out all breads, pastas, sugary products, fruit (with the exception of the occasional raspberry or blueberry or strawberry in very limited quantity). Meat and protein consumption needs to be limited as well, since consuming an over-abundance in protein will cause the protein products to be broken down into glucose for processing. This takes us out of the ketogenic state, and we don't get that fat burning we are going for.

Before starting the diet, you will want to clear out all of the high-carb foods you have on hand. Give the foods away, donate them or give them to co-workers and friends. (This is healthier than having one last starchy meal before beginning). Buy a scale and other measuring tools so you can keep constant tabs on what you are consuming. This is important to maintaining the ketones in the body. Another convenient tool are keto-stix, which measure the presence of ketones in urine.

There are also more expensive, yet more effective tools on the market for measuring the actual amount of ketones in the blood, and these require the drawing of blood. You can do this in the comfort of your home (but it's also good to keep in touch with your doctor if you are unsure at any point).

The advantage with checking the ketones in the blood is you get to see just how many ketones there really are. When you look at the presence of ketones in the urine, you don't see how many you are absorbing through the kidneys (since you are just peeing them out). As time goes by, and you have been on the diet after a week and more, the body will increasingly become more effective at absorbing ketones and using them for energy. A blood test will reflect this better than a urine test. Still, the keto-stix are available at your local drugstore and online shops such as Amazon, and this is an easy way to get some picture of whether you are in the ketogenic state or not.

Chapter 3:
Fat, Fat, Fat

Did you know that fat is actually really good for you? (Ok, not trans-fat, or hydrogenated oils, they are still bad). Fat is good for the brain, and pregnant women are recommended to get plenty of good fat like coconut oil.

On the ketogenic diet, you will also want to focus on getting lots of fat in your diet. Bacon? No problem. Save that bacon grease to fry foods in later. It's good for you (really, I promise). Tons of butter? Great! A spoonful of coconut oil with your breakfast? Excellent idea! Go for it.

What you need to watch out for is first and foremost carbohydrates since they halt the production of ketones and ketones in your body are what you want. Protein can also have the same effect if too much of it is eaten. A tiny bit of certain items containing a little carbs are OK (we'll show you which ones later on in this book). Some protein is also good for you, especially when there's a lot of fat along with it. We'll also help you figure that one out.

An average value for daily-consumed nutrients is 136 grams of fat, 74 grams of protein, and 20 grams of net carbs from a 1600 calorie a day diet plan. As you can see, this is a lot of fat, a decent amount of protein, and a really small value for carbs. The next thing to address here are what are "net carbs"? Net carbs are the amount of carbohydrates one eats, minus fiber. So if you are eating something with 10 grams of carbohydrates, but it also has 2 grams of fiber, take away the grams of fiber and you have 8 net grams of carbs to count toward your daily values.

The amounts given above are an average for women who don't work out very much, so if you're either an athlete, go to the gym pretty often, or a large man, you can adjust these values a bit to increase them accordingly (but the ratio of 4:1 fat vs. carbs and protein, 75% fat, 20% protein and 5% carbohydrates needs to be maintained in order for the diet to work.)

Make it Pure Fat...

So if you want to fill up on something, make it pure fat. A spoonful of organic coconut oil is great. Add an extra serving of butter to your steak. Chicken fat in your soup broth (homemade bone broth is especially healthy, and good for digestion). This is where you are allowed to go wild. But by no means can you allow yourself to "cheat". Off days, or off meals, or even one serving too many carbs will throw you out of the ketogenic state and then you will start over from scratch. The point is to maintain the diet, and to keep it over an extended period to optimize the benefits. (The body will absorb the ketones better and better over time, you need to have patience and dedication to get yourself there!) Also, remember to not overdo it on the proteins as they are converted to glucose (sugar) when you eat too much. This means you need to stick to the portions given in the recipes, when in doubt.

In western (American, European) society, we grow up thinking fat is the enemy and grains (especially whole grains) are good for us. In fact, it's the opposite. (Though you do still want to avoid hydrogenated fats). For this reason, it's helpful to adhere exactly to recipes, shopping lists while strictly measuring out portions. We don't want to fall back into old ways of thinking and habits regarding our eating.

Chapter 4:
Who Should Go on the Ketogenic Diet?

If you're uncertain if this diet is for you, consult your doctor. The diet is good for most people who have spent most of their lives eating too many carbs. It's good for those of us who have had a hard time getting that 10 pounds off, despite the many diets we've tried over the years, and hard training at the gym.

Some conditions that do not allow for this diet are pancreatitis, abnormal liver function, gall bladder problems, the inability to digest fat, carnitine deficiency, poor nutritional status (as in the inability to absorb nutrients). Talk to your doctor and find out if any of these or other conditions apply to you.(This is not an expansive list, so make sure you talk to a professional before starting this or other diets).

Studies have found that the ketogenic diet improves sociability, mood and functioning among people with autism. Some lab tests done with mice showed the same results. Epileptic seizures in those with epilepsy disappear over time, if the diet is maintained. People with multiple sclerosis have reported great results. The high fat diet reduces inflammation of tissues in the body. Inflammation causes a great deal of stress and manifests as pain in sufferers of MS. The diet also prevents cell damage which is of aid to everyone, particularly those with serious illness.

In the elderly, the ketogenic diet has been employed to slow the onset of those genetically pre-disposed to Alzheimer's disease. Cell damage is one of the reasons for the disease, and the diet prevents this. The diet is considered to possess a neuro-protective effect, which hinders neurological damage associated with the conditions mentioned above. Studies have shown the ketogenic diet to help heal and mitigate damage with Parkinson's disease, brain injury and stroke. The body is able to regenerate, or at least further degeneration is prevented allowing healing mechanisms to do their work. The fatty acids which are released into the liver when ketones are present contribute to the oxidation of triglycerides. The specific ketone thought to be responsible for this is β-hydroxybutyrate.

Studies also showed, of note that even one meal high in carbohydrates caused all positive effects to disappear.

Personal anecdotes reveal that many people believe the ketogenic diet also can help people who are undergoing cancer treatment. The cancer cells are effectively stunted in their growth, so that when medical professionals apply their mode of treatment it takes less time to get the cancer under control.

Academic articles and studies on the topic are skeptical to the diet as far as the successful administration of it. In other words, their tends to be doubts as to getting adult patients prescribed by their doctors to stick to the diet. Other than that, studies are full of positive results in treating a whole slew of illnesses, particularly neurological disorders. This should be motivation for those of us who take to the diet of our own free will. We can prevent the onset of these diseases; keep ourselves fit, possibly cancer-free, and strong of mind and body.

Chapter 5:
Foods to Eat, Foods to Avoid

These are some of the delicious foods you can enjoy on this healthful diet.

- Think large amounts of butter, slathered over a decent-sized, delicious cut of steak
- A crispy green salad with lots of olives and olive oil, avocado and two strips of bacon or a piece of chicken
- Full-fat Greek yoghurt for breakfast
- A ketogenic vanilla smoothie
- Almond flour low carb bread.
- So much more!

What you absolutely shouldn't consume on the keto diet:

Alcohol - Alcohol is devoid of nutrition, and breaks down as sugar. It also stresses the liver. One glass and you start over from square one. Avoid it.

"Low-carb"candies - These sweets are usually processed, and contain maltodextrin, dextrose and other junk, which breaks down as glucose in the body.

Tropical fruit - This means mangos, bananas, pineapples, papayas. They are high in sugar.

Dried fruit - The amount of sugar becomes more concentrated when fruits are dried. Avoid raisins, figs, etc.

Milk - (Cream, sour cream, cheese, and high-fat yoghurt are all OK) The milk that is generally available has been heated to the point where the pasteurization kills off gut-friendly bacteria. It is also high in sugar.

Grains - Don't order that pizza. The crust is bread; you want to avoid it and its ilk. This means rice, quinoa, whole wheat, buckwheat, corn meal, potatoes, millet, barley are all out. You won't miss them once you've lost that weight you've always tried to kick to the curb, but couldn't. (Think: no food tastes as good as the sweet feeling of success in having achieved your ideal weight.)

Processed Foods - Avoiding pre-packaged foods will make your life easier. Why? You don't have to bother figuring out whether some hidden ingredient will throw off your diet. The additives and the methods which are used to make such items are not always clear. Besides, you want to stick to real, whole foods which will give you the nutrition you need to be the best you, you can be.

Corn - Avoid all corn and corn products. Corn causes inflammation, is starchy and is metabolized as glucose. Besides, it is usually genetically modified and that's extremely unhealthy to consume.

What's OK in Moderation:

Berries. A few blueberries, raspberries, strawberries, blackberries, currants, nectarine, apple, cherries, plums, watermelon, cantaloupe, grapes, fresh figs, peaches are all OK in very small amounts. Don't overdo it. For best results, allow yourself a green apple in your smoothie every once in awhile.

Root vegetables. (Vegetables that grows underground) Rutabaga, parsnip, sweet potato, carrot, beets are OK in limited amounts. They have some starch, so this counts toward your carbohydrate intake. You will want to find out how many carbs are in each of these vegetables so you can keep track.

Nuts. Nuts such as macadamia are great because they are very high in healthy fats. Still, you don't want to go overboard. Others, such as peanuts should be eaten only very sparingly. Hazelnuts, cashews, pine nuts, pistachios, walnuts, almonds can also be eaten in moderation and are a source of natural fat. A handful here and there is a tasty and healthy snack.

Milk products and cheese. Go for full fat milk products such as cream, sour cream and cheese. Don't consume these to excess since they do contain protein and carbohydrates, besides fat. Cheeses like mozzarella, ricotta, brie, cheddar, camembert, parmesan, etc. are delicious and can be enjoyed in moderation.

Seeds. Flax seeds, pumpkin seeds, and sunflower seeds are OK to eat here and there. Sunflower seed butter is also available some places, or you can make your own. Sunflower seeds can be ground up in a coffee grinder to yield a flour-like consistency. Add oil, salt and spices and roll them up into a ball for an easy snack. (Read on for more recipes and tips later on in this book).

Spices and seasonings. You want your food to taste good, so feel free to use spices and seasonings (natural source). However, basil, oregano, garlic, turmeric, cilantro, cinnamon, black pepper, cayenne pepper, sage, rosemary, thyme and so forth do contain carbohydrates, so you need to count these toward your daily limit. As far as salt is concerned, choose sea salt or ayurveda salt (the pretty pink salt) since these are more nutritious with minerals still present and are not cut with dextrin and other not OK products (like typical "table salt" is).

Meat and fish. Meat and fish count toward protein, which we have to remember counts toward starch in the body if too much is eaten. So we can enjoy fish filets and steak sometimes, but in limited amounts. For example, 2 strips of bacon is allowed. (Each piece contains 2.9 grams of protein, 0 carbs, 3.5 grams of fat) Chicken, beef, fish, ham, tuna, salmon, turkey, shrimp, scallops, crab, lobster, lamb, veal, cod are all OK. Don't exceed portions given in recipes, or else the body could stop producing the ketones needed to maintain the state of fat burning as an energy source. Most things that walk on land or swim in the sea are completely OK to eat on the ketogenic diet. Go for organic wherever possible, for optimal health.

Things to eat more of:

Low carbohydrate vegetables. Go for vegetables that are green and leafy, and grow above ground. They are full of vitamins, minerals and low in carbs. Asparagus is delicious and healthy. Lettuce of all types is the perfect accompanying some high fat item, and a bit of meat. Avocado is not only low carb, but high in healthy fat. Celery is refreshing, crispy and a great choice of vegetable. Onions and green beans are ok in moderation. Broccoli and cauliflower are fine to eat. Cucumber and tomatoes are a good addition to a salad. Squash and shallots can be cooked and eaten in a little soup. Pay attention to portions and don't go overboard.

Oils and fats. Use natural oils and fats to cook your food. This includes butter, ghee (Indian clarified butter), olive oil, beef tallow, coconut oil, coconut butter, mayonnaise (be sure there isn't any added sugar of any kind, including agave syrup in which case you cannot use it), red palm oil, chicken fat, bacon fat, and other types of natural fats of plant and animal sources. If there are no carbs at all in your choice of oil or fat, feel free to take an extra portion to go with your meal. (Make sure you double-check this).

Water. Drink lots and lots of water. People on the ketogenic diet tend to need to use the bathroom a lot, due to the ketones not being absorbed as efficiently in the beginning of the diet. It gets better over time, but it's important to drink enough water particularly when you start out. Once you get in the habit of always having a glass or a bottle of water with you at every second of the day, you might as well continue. Drinking enough water ensures that impurities in the body can safely leave via the urine. It makes more work for the body to expel toxins out the skin, so drinking enough water is always a good idea for health and wellness.

Herbal tea. Drink herbal tea and decaf coffee. Choose organic herbal tea wherever possible. Many of them have health-giving properties all their own. For example, peppermint is calming to the stomach. Chamomile and lavender promote restful sleep. Stinging nettle tea is good for the skin. Decaf coffee is a good option for those who love the taste of coffee and don't want to sacrifice this pastime.

What About Caffeine?

Regarding caffeine and the ketogenic diet: Some say caffeine in tea and coffee during the ketogenic diet is OK. Others say it is an absolute no-go because it impairs the impact of the ketones. Studies don't reveal any evidence in either direction. If you want to be sure that your diet is effective, don't cut corners and take any chances on anything, including the topic of caffeine. The strictest diets exclude coffee.

The candida diet, which is very similar to the ketogenic diet excludes coffee and caffeinated tea because of the effects it has on the adrenals. The caffeine causes the adrenals to pump out adrenaline, which causes a temporary feeling of alertness. The strain on the adrenals, the heart and nervous system this causes is said to be detrimental to health. If you are on the ketogenic diet to lose weight and improve your health, the best you can do is to cut out caffeine and enjoy herbal tea and decaf coffee.

Another aspect of this controversy is the part insulin resistance plays. Insulin resistance is lowered on the ketogenic diet because ketones improve insulin sensitivity, thus making it possible for cells to more easily absorb glucose. It is thought that caffeine interferes with this process and thus disrupts the diet. It is your choice, but it is another reason to avoid caffeine when on the ketogenic diet.

Sweeteners and the Ketogenic Diet: Artificial sweeteners such as xylitol, Splenda and the like should be avoided particularly in powder form as they are cut with corn byproducts. They also contain carbs. The best artificial sweetener is stevia, which is a plant that is naturally sweet and devoid of carbs. Find it in liquid form and add it to your tea, full-fat Greek yoghurt and ketogenic-approved desserts. (Some recipes included in this book). To sum it up: **liquid stevia** is the best choice for a sweetener; don't bother with the others as there is typically some carbohydrate-related drawback to consider. You can buy liquid stevia online, at health food shops and even some standard supermarkets.

Chapter 6:
Delicious and Healthy Ketogenic Recipes

Here's the chapter for practical application of the ketogenic diet. Here is where you get to try out something new and good to get your body burning fat. This is the place to really start when you are ready to make a diet overhaul to totally renew and rejuvenate your body, possibly slow cancer growth or prevent it, protect your brain and nervous system, and lose plenty of unwanted weight! Here you will find easy and practical recipes for breakfast, lunch, dinner, dessert, snacks and smoothies. You will have fun trying out these recipes and getting on the road to better health fast. Enjoy!

Easy and Sweet Breakfast Yogurt

Ingredients:

- A cup of fage (or another type of Greek yoghurt) full fat yoghurt
- A few drops of liquid stevia (vanilla flavor is delicious!)
- A few almonds, or a pinch of shredded coconut to top

Directions:

Scoop the yoghurt into a bowl. Add a few drops of stevia and stir. (Go easy on the stevia, it's really powerful and it's not hard to accidentally add too much of it. A little really goes a long way) Top the breakfast treat with a few almonds or another type of nut of your choice. A pinch of shredded coconut is also a tasty way to liven up this quick and easy breakfast. It really is delicious, so easy and you can also eat it as a snack any time of the day. (Just be careful to not eat too much, the yoghurt does have protein. One cup a day is the maximum amount allowed)

Bread? Why not? (Ketogenic approved, of course)

The breakfast rolls below are pretty simple to make. You can double the amount and freeze some rolls for later use. You can eat one for breakfast, or for lunch with cold cuts and butter. Top with sugar-free tomato paste and cheese for a pizza roll. You can pack them and take them to work with you to eat at your desk. They are good enough to offer to guests. The consistency is great and they are delicious simply with butter, but with cream cheese they are a real delight!

Ketogenic Breakfast Rolls

Ingredients:

- 1.5 cups Almond flour (purchase as is, or grind almonds in a coffee grinder to make your own)
- Two thirds of a cup of powdered psyllium husk
- .5 cup coconut flour (make your own by putting shredded coconut into a food processor and processing it into flour consistency. This is much better and cheaper than the store bought variety)
- .5 cup flaxseed meal (grind golden or brown flax seeds in a coffee grinder, or purchase flaxseed meal at a health food store)
- 2 teaspoons of cream of tartar
- 2 teaspoons of garlic and/or onion powder
- 1 teaspoon of baking powder
- 1 teaspoon of sea salt
- Seeds for topping the finished rolls
- 6-7 egg whites
- 2 eggs
- 2 cups of warm water

How to make the rolls:

1. Preheat oven to 350 degrees Fahrenheit.
2. Mix the dry ingredients except for the powdered psyllium husk and the seeds in a bowl.
3. Mix the psyllium powder in a separate bowl with the egg whites, the 2 eggs and the 2 cups of warm water.
4. Combine the two bowls into one and mix using a hand mixer.
5. When the ingredients are well combined, form rolls using your hands and a spoon. Sprinkle the rolls with your choice of seeds (sesame, pumpkin, sunflower etc)
6. Place them on a baking sheet with parchment paper leaving enough space between the rolls since they will rise and expand.
7. Bake for 45 minutes. Remove the rolls and allow to cool. Top them with butter and eat on the go, or make sandwiches with a bit of bacon, turkey, cheese, lettuce. Enjoy!

Ketogenic Green Smoothie

Green smoothies give you a boost in the morning as a breakfast, or are a healthful mid day meal or snack. This one is particularly full of veggie- goodness and greens. It is super low on carbohydrates. (Green apples are among the lowest carb of the low carb fruits) Get your vitamins the healthy and yummy way!

Ingredients:

- A cup of carrageenan free, unsweetened almond milk
- Half an avocado
- A green apple, peeled and cut into bits to make processing easier
- A handful of spinach
- A few drops of liquid stevia

Directions:

Fill a magic bullet blender cup with the avocado, green apple bits and spinach. Pour in the almond milk. If desired, you can add some water and ice cubes to the mix. Add a couple drops of stevia in blend. For a protein boost, add a scoop of organic peanut butter or organic almond butter, or even better: macadamia butter. To increase your veggie intake, add a couple slices of cucumber. Enjoy!

Ketogenic Vanilla Smoothie

Here's an easy and really fast recipe for meals on the go, or for snacks and desserts. Add a couple raspberries or blueberries for a fruity, yet low-carb experience. Real vanilla makes this delicious and enjoyable.

Ingredients:

- 2 cups full fat Greek yoghurt (preferably organic)
- Vanilla powder (pure, without additives) or real vanilla scraped from a vanilla pod (recommended)
- A few drops of Stevia

Directions:

Pour all of the ingredients into a blender. Blend until smooth. Enjoy in a glass in the sun, or on the way to work for a fast and nourishing breakfast.

Ketogenic Pancakes

This recipe for pancakes doesn't even use flour, so you can enjoy with a good conscience. They are so simple to make, so good to eat, and versatile. (Try them on the go as a type of wrap to put cheese or meat or avocado in as a type of wrap sandwich). You can eat them for breakfast or dessert, or be creative and use them as a part of another meal. Cinnamon, ginger, vanilla, cocoa are all great to give these a little kick.

Ingredients:

- 2 eggs
- 2 ounces of cream cheese
- A few drops of liquid stevia
- Vanilla from a vanilla powder or a pinch of cinnamon
- Butter for frying

Directions:

Blend the 2 eggs and the cream cheese. Add the stevia and the spices. Blend until smooth. Heat and melt the butter in the frying pan. Once the pan is hot, pour a pancake-sized amount of batter into the frying pan. Once the sides are firm enough to flip (this should take about two minutes), flip the pancake and let it cook for another minute or until a nice golden brown color. Enjoy with a bit of sour cream and/or a couple of berries (such as strawberries sliced, blueberries, or raspberries, or blackberries, etc.).

Homemade Almond Milk

Almond milk can be purchased everywhere these days. You can even find it unsweetened. However, a lot of processed additives can throw you off course with your diet. The best thing you can do is to make your own yummy and fresh almond milk. It's really easy, but requires a blender, cheesecloth and a bowl.

Ingredients:

- 2 cups of organic pre-soaked almonds
- 5-6 cups of water

Directions:

Soak the almonds in a clean bowl with water for 5 hours. Rinse the almonds until the water runs clear. (This takes away any anti-nutrients in the water, from the almonds) Pour in the water. Process in the blender until you see the water has become almond milk. Place the cheesecloth over the top of the blender and pour the resulting almond milk into a pitcher or large class of your choosing. You can even use the almond meal resulting in recipes calling for almond flour. The almond milk you have made can now be enjoyed. Add some vanilla powder or stevia drops to sweeten and add flavor. (Also cinnamon, cocoa, etc can be added for a delicious and easy treat).

Easy Ketogenic Lunch Salad

This salad is easy to prepare, and great to enjoy.

Ingredients:

- Two cups of lettuce
- One tomato, chopped
- One quarter of a cucumber, sliced
- Half an avocado sliced or chopped
- One slice of bacon, fried
- Half a hard boiled egg
- Olive oil to top
- A pinch of salt and pepper to season

Directions:

Chop all vegetables as desired. Fry some bacon. (Refrigerate the slices you don't use) Boil some eggs. Use half of a peeled egg for this salad, save the others for later. Top the salad with a generous amount of olive oil. Sprinkle with salt and pepper and a small amount of other herbs if so desired. Eat the salad right away, or pack and consume on the go.

Delicious, Hearty Dinner Recipes

The next recipe makes for a wonderful, hearty and filling dinner or big lunch on the weekend. It's deliciously cheesy, full of fat and healthy broccoli and is super easy to make! You need a casserole dish, a stove and an oven to make it, besides the listed ingredients below.

Cheesy Broccoli Chicken Bake

Ingredients:

- 1 head of broccoli
- Quarter of a stick of butter for frying
- 1 chicken breast
- 1 green bell pepper
- 1 yellow onion
- 2 cloves of garlic.
- 6 strips bacon
- 8 ounces shredded cheddar cheese
- 8 ounces shredded mozzarella
- 8 ounces cream cheese
- 4 ounces full fat cream

Procedure:

1. Fry the bacon on the stovetop. Put the butter into another pan and fry the chicken over the stovetop. Dice the pepper, onion and garlic. Chop the broccoli into nice bite-size florets.
2. Preheat the oven to 350 degrees Fahrenheit.
3. Add the pepper, onion and garlic to the chicken once it is nearly cooked through, in the same pan and fry them. Cut the chicken into strips and continue to fry.
4. Lightly steam the broccoli. Place in the casserole dish. Add the chicken, peppers, onions and garlic and stir to combine. Add the cream cheese, the cream and half of the mozzarella and cheddar and stir all of these together.
5. Top the casserole with the other half of the mozzarella and cheddar.
6. Bake for 30 minutes.
7. Enjoy with a small green salad on the side. Serves 2 people.

Easy Ketogenic Dinner

Ingredients:

- One salmon filet (if frozen, allow the filet to defrost over a few hours)
- An onion
- A clove of garlic
- A lemon
- Butter for frying (or ghee, olive oil, or coconut oil)
- Baby spinach greens
- A quarter of a cucumber
- Some asparagus tops
- Olive oil
- Salt and pepper

Procedure:

1. Chop the onion and the garlic.
2. Put the salmon in a frying pan with the butter. Fry on medium heat until the salmon is almost entirely cooked through. Add the chopped onion and garlic to the pan and fry together until the salmon is entirely cooked through.

3. Toss the spinach greens, cucumber and asparagus tops in a bowl with the olive oil and the salt and pepper. Squeeze a bit of lemon onto the salad.

4. Serve the salmon on the salad. Squeeze a bit of lemon juice over the salmon as well.

   Enjoy!

Simple Ketogenic Snacks

Here are two easy recipes that involve just a few ingredients. They are easy for beginners to the diet, as well as people who don't have much experience in the kitchen. They will hardly take any of your time, but will leave you feeling satisfied.

Cucumber, cold cut and Cheese Rolls

Ingredients:

- 2 thin slices of cucumber, cut lengthwise using a mandolin or a vegetable peeler
- 2 pieces of cold cut meat (ham, turkey, chicken etc)
- 2 pieces of cheddar

Directions:

Assemble a slice of cucumber with a piece of cold cut meat and a piece of cheddar. Roll them together. Repeat the process with the other pieces and eat on the go.

Avocado Egg

(Makes for a delicious breakfast, lunch or dinner or snack)

Ingredients:

- 2 eggs
- 1 avocado
- A bit of salt and pepper
- Some butter for frying the eggs

Directions:

Fry an egg over the stove with some butter. Slice the avocado in half, remove the pit and place the fried egg where the pit was. Repeat with the other egg and avocado half. Season with a bit of salt and pepper. Bon appétit! Serves 1 person.

Ketogenic Desserts

Just because you are on a diet that is extremely efficient at burning fat and strict to maintain, doesn't mean you can't enjoy dessert... (Very low carb, sugar free dessert that is)

Here are two types of pudding. One is even vegan and lactose-free. Both are delicious and extremely easy to make.

Keto Chocolate Pudding (Milk based)

Ingredients:

- 6 ounces of cream cheese
- 5 ounces of whipping cream
- A few drops of liquid stevia
- A few spoonful's of pure cocoa powder

Directions:

Mix all of the ingredients with a hand mixer until smooth and a pudding consistency has been achieved. Serves 2 people.

Keto Almond Chia Pudding

Ingredients:

- 3 heaping Tablespoons chia seeds
- 1 cup unsweetened almond milk
- A few drops stevia
- A spoonful of almond butter

Directions:

Put the chia seeds into a bowl. Add the almond milk and stir. When the chia seeds and almond milk have achieved a pudding-like consistency, add the stevia drops and stir well. Top with a bit of almond butter.

Here's a creamy, dreamy smoothie to enjoy as a dessert. You can't taste the spinach or the avocado, but they make the consistency creamy and smooth.

Raspberry Cocoa Dream Smoothie

Ingredients:

- Half an avocado
- A handful of raspberries
- A good handful of baby spinach
- 2 cups unsweetened almond milk
- 3 drops of stevia
- 2 tablespoons full of cocoa powder
- A tablespoonful of peanut butter

Directions:

Put all of the ingredients into a blender and blend until all of the ingredients are well combined. You can taste test the smoothie and decide whether to add a drop or two more of stevia, if you'd like to have it a bit sweeter. Can also be enjoyed for breakfast.

Blueberry Ketogenic Muffins

A delicious treat for dessert or breakfast. Enjoy it with plenty of butter, or coconut oil on top.

Ingredients:

- 2 cups of almond meal
- 1 teaspoon baking soda
- A few drops of lemon extract
- 1 cup of full fat cream
- 2-3 eggs
- ½ stick of melted butter
- A few drops of stevia
- A handful of blueberries

Procedure:

1. Preheat your oven to 350 degrees Fahrenheit.
2. Combine the dry ingredients (the almond flour and the baking soda)
3. Then add the cream and mix with a hand mixer.
4. Then add the eggs one at a time and mix. (If the mixture is smooth but not too runny, there's no need to use all three eggs, but if the mixture seems too thick, go ahead and add another egg).
5. Add the drops of stevia and lemon extract and mix.

6. Fold in the blueberries carefully to the batter.

7. Pour the mixture into muffin cups so the cups are halfway full in a muffin pan and bake for about 25 minutes, or until the muffins are a golden brown.

   Tip: use raspberries or strawberries instead of blueberries for variation. A yummy topping might also be almond or macadamia butter.

With these and other delicious ketogenic diet recipes, you won't miss starches and sweets. These muffins, smoothies, rolls, dinners, filling salads and other delicious dishes are better than the "standard" diet. They're also a whole lot healthier! No need to hold the butter!

Chapter 7:
Tips and Inspiration

No diet is easy. No lifestyle change is easy. However, if the diet and the lifestyle change mean amazing health, increased metabolism, weight loss, controlling inflammation, stopping seizures, improved skin tone (acne control), treating multiple diseases, then it's well worth it. We can also infer that the ketogenic diet helps against migraines, since migraines and other forms of pain in the body are caused by inflammation, and the diet gets inflammation under control, or eliminates it entirely. Sufferers of chronic back pain and sciatica have also had great results under the diet. Some even claim to get colds less, or not at all, after having gone on the diet. The immune system is better equipped to handle the outside world.

On the ketogenic diet, you are allowed 136 grams of fat, 74 grams of protein, and 20 grams of net carbs from a 1600 calorie a day. This is the right proportion to keep your body in ketosis (using fat for fuel instead of glucose). If you train a lot, then you may adjust this to a slightly higher amount while maintaining the proportions of 75% fat, 20% protein and 5% carbohydrates. (You can find macronutrient calculators on the internet which allow you to input your weight, height and activity level. The amounts specified here are a good average for women)

You need to stick with a diet plan and adhere to it to keep your body's glucose levels low enough to produce the wanted ketones. You can't have one off-meal, or all of the beneficial effects will disappear at once. (As studies showed with patients of epilepsy: one non-ketogenic meal and their seizures returned and they had to start over again). If you go off the diet, you will have to start from square one because it takes time for the glucose in the body to be released and used up. Only when that has occurred is it possible for ketones to be produced and used as an energy source. So stick with it!

It also helps to exercise, especially when you start the diet since this will help get the glucose in the body used up and the ketones getting produced and absorbed faster.

When starting the diet, some people report feeling tired and moody. This is normal, and it helps to exercise and to drink lots of water to improve your mood. Herbal teas like St. John's wort can also help elevate your mood. Whatever you do to mitigate this phase, it will be over before you know it and you will feel better than ever.

Try a bone broth soup and try adding a little more salt than usual to your food to help prevent excessive water loss.

Needing to go to the bathroom more than usual is also totally normal. Drink lots of water, and get plenty of salt. Take a liquid magnesium supplement and try a magnesium oil spray to replenish nutrients. Your body will adjust soon enough, and in the meantime you can help it out by getting plenty of rest, exercising moderately and taking some supplements, and drinking lots of water.

For social support, do an online search for forums to talk to others who are also trying the ketogenic diet. There are sure to be people who can provide moral support, offer their wisdom and knowledge.

After a week of the diet, it gets much easier. If you adhere to the diet strictly, the tough phase will be over faster and it will become second nature. Easy as (ketogenic diet friendly) pie.

You can do it!

Conclusion

Sugar is highly overrated. The body doesn't need it to function normally. In fact, sugar is a detriment to health. We can run on fat instead of sugar, and this is the better way. The body is able to control inflammation, lower the risk of diseases such as cancer, stop pain, stop acne, drop pounds, help brain function, help slow Alzheimer's disease, stop premature aging, prevent colds, stop the flu... the list goes on and on. The only thing we have to do to get these benefits is to make some simple diet adjustments.

As simple as these adjustments are, they require will power and the ability to commit to a lifestyle change. You can't just start up the diet and stop after two days: that's not enough to reap any sort of positive transformation You need to get on the diet and plan in at least a month to begin to notice any changes. At best, you will get on the diet and never go off, since the benefits to the health are so numerous and all encompassing.

Medical studies have been conducted that even found the ketogenic diet to help autism. There are so many aspects of life that this diet can change for the better. It's not pseudo-science or speculation: doctors found as early as the 1920's that the ketogenic diet can put a stop to seizures.

The diet was rediscovered in the 90's, and since then, thousands of people have used the diet to transform their lives.

Ketones are metabolic units that are produced in the body when glucose levels fall. The body is then able to use fat to burn as energy, and stored fat disappears from the body, as the liver is able to process this.

Ketones can help us to finally achieve our ideal weight, to stop our back pain, to stop migraines, have great skin, and to live the lives we want! Those who maintain the diet all report success; you can have this success too! We wish you the best of luck! Have fun enjoying your newfound health! This is really the best thing you can do for yourself.

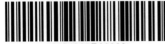

12154385R00033

Printed in Great Britain
by Amazon.co.uk, Ltd.,
Marston Gate.